DEFEATING HYPERTENSION WITH EXPERT GUIDANCE

Ultimate Solution Handbook For Patients, Guardians Or Family To Understand, Manage, Treat, Prevent, Reverse Symptoms And Live Well

DR. POTTER WHITLEY

DISCLAIMER:

This book's contents are meant to be used solely for informative purposes. The information should not be used as a replacement for expert medical advice, diagnosis, or care.

The information contained in this book is accurate and reliable, having been verified by the author to the best of his ability. Nevertheless, the author disclaims all express and implied representations and warranties regarding the availability, correctness, appropriateness, completeness, and reliability of the material provided here. You bear full responsibility for any reliance you may have on such material.

For informational purposes, this book may make reference to or mention of certain people, things, websites, organizations, or other names. The author has no connection to, endorsement from, or recommendation for these organizations. The author's approval or validation is not implied by the inclusion of these references.

Any direct, indirect, incidental, special, or consequential damages resulting from using or not being able to use the material in this book are not covered by the author's liability policy. For medical advice and counsel particular to their circumstances, readers are advised to check with experienced healthcare specialists.

The content, materials, and information in this book are subject to change at any time without prior notice, at the author's discretion. The text may contain errors or omissions for which the author is not responsible.

By reading this book, you understand and accept the conditions of this disclaimer.

THE REASON BEHIND THIS BOOK

"Defeating HYPERTENSION With Expert Guidance" is a valuable resource in the field of health literature that provides an in-depth analysis of hypertension, a disorder that impacts millions of people globally. The first section of the book takes the reader through the complexities of hypertension, explaining what it is and emphasizing how important it is to control blood pressure. It skillfully draws attention to the risk factors linked to hypertension, promoting a thorough awareness that enables readers to take charge of their health.

After skimming the surface, the book delves into blood pressure physiology, explaining how the body uses it. The author fills in the information vacuum by focusing on the subtle differences between normal and high blood pressure and making the connection between these physiological details and their wider effects on cardiovascular health. This basic understanding lays the groundwork for readers to understand the silent dangers of asymptomatic hypertension, identify signs, and decide whether to seek medical assistance.

This book is exceptional since it is dedicated to real-world solutions. Readers are educated about the significance of exercise, stress management strategies, and a balanced diet in the section on lifestyle adjustments. This all-encompassing method acknowledges the relationship between different aspects of life and how it affects blood pressure. The book also informs readers about the variety of hypertension drugs available, including complementary therapies, and stresses the combination of medicine and lifestyle modifications.

This guide's emphasis on giving people the tools they need to take control of their health at home is one of its best features. With tips on selecting the best blood pressure monitor, keeping up regular monitoring, and interpreting readings, it demystifies the process of controlling blood pressure. The book emphasizes the value of routine examinations and the cooperative relationship between patients and healthcare providers.

With special sections on the effects of hypertension on the heart and kidneys, as well as its connections to diabetes and other illnesses, the complex relationship between hypertension and other medical diseases is expertly examined. In addition, the book offers helpful advice on dietary strategies, supporting the well-known DASH diet and providing dietary guidelines and preparation instructions for heart-healthy meals.

Beyond the short-term difficulties, the manual explores the psychological elements of managing hypertension. It discusses typical roadblocks, promotes the development of a strong support network, and offers advice on sustaining motivation over the long term. To serve as a resource for the future, the book finishes by examining potential developments and trends in the management of hypertension, such as advancements in medical research, the use of technology in blood pressure monitoring, and innovative approaches to prevention.

"Defeating HYPERTENSION With Expert Guidance" essentially goes beyond the bounds of conventional health literature. This comprehensive guide provides readers with the necessary knowledge, resources, and inspiration to successfully manage the intricate world of hypertension. It not only guarantees immediate well-being but also a future filled with proactive health decisions.

TABLE OF CONTENT

CHAPTER ONE

INTRODUCTION TO HYPERTENSION
What Is Elevated Blood Pressure?

Elevated blood pressure within the arteries is the hallmark of hypertension, also referred to as high blood pressure. The force that the blood exerts on the artery walls as the heart pumps blood throughout the body is known as blood pressure. It is expressed as the difference between the systolic and diastolic pressures and is measured in millimeters of mercury (mmHg). The force experienced by the heart during a beat is represented by the diastolic pressure, whereas the force during a systolic beat is that of the heart at rest.

Typically, normal blood pressure is 120/80 mmHg. When these readings continuously rise above the normal range, which is commonly defined as 130/80 mmHg or higher, hypertension results. It's a chronic illness that can cause serious health problems like kidney damage, heart disease, and stroke if ignored.

Hypertension is caused by several variables, including underlying medical disorders, lifestyle decisions, and heredity. The most prevalent kind of hypertension, known as primary hypertension, is causeless and develops gradually over time. Kidney illness or hormonal imbalances are examples of underlying conditions that lead to secondary hypertension. Regular blood pressure monitoring is essential for the early detection and treatment of hypertension because the condition is frequently asymptomatic in its early stages.

The Value of Blood Pressure Management

It's critical to effectively control blood pressure to preserve general health and avoid possibly fatal consequences. Elevated blood pressure increases the risk of cardiovascular diseases by placing stress on the heart, arteries, and other organs. Atherosclerosis, a disorder where arteries constrict and harden and impede blood flow, can be brought on over time by continuous strain on arterial walls.

Lifestyle changes and sometimes medication are necessary for blood pressure control. A heart-healthy diet, regular exercise, keeping a healthy weight, cutting back on alcohol, and giving up smoking are a few examples of lifestyle modifications. These actions improve general well-being in addition to lowering blood pressure.

Those with severe hypertension or those who are at high risk of consequences may require medical measures. Physicians administer antihypertensive drugs to control blood pressure and lessen the heart's workload. Adherence to medication, frequent monitoring, and follow-ups with healthcare providers are essential elements of effective blood pressure management.

Risk Factors for High Blood Pressure

It is crucial to comprehend the risk factors linked to hypertension to avoid and treat the condition early on. A person can alter some risk factors by lifestyle modifications, but not all of them are within their control. Age, family history, and race are non-modifiable risk variables; people of African origin, for instance, are more likely to have hypertension.

Poor food choices, a sedentary lifestyle, being overweight, smoking, consuming too much alcohol, and high-stress levels are examples of modifiable risk factors. High-sodium, low-potassium diets are especially associated with high blood pressure.

People can drastically lower their risk of acquiring hypertension by addressing modifiable risk factors. As was previously indicated, lifestyle changes are essential for prevention. In addition to avoiding tobacco and excessive alcohol use, maintaining a healthy blood pressure level and delaying the onset of hypertension-related problems can be achieved by regular exercise, a balanced diet, stress management, and other lifestyle choices. For people who are at risk, routine blood pressure checks and physical examinations are crucial for early identification and prompt management.

CHAPTER TWO

THE PHYSIOLOGY OF BLOOD PRESSURE
The Mechanism of Blood Pressure:

A crucial physiological indicator, blood pressure gauges the force of blood on artery walls as the heart pumps blood throughout the body. This force is essential for providing tissues and organs with nutrition and oxygen. Systolic pressure, or the force the heart applies to the artery walls during a contraction, and diastolic pressure, or the force the heart exerts between beats, are the two numbers that are commonly used to express blood pressure. Millimeters of mercury (mmHg) are used as the unit of measurement.

During the systolic phase, the heart pumps blood into the arteries with great force. The higher numerical number of blood pressure readings is produced by this force. The lower numerical value is then produced by the heart relaxing during the diastolic phase, which results in a pressure drop. To ensure that organs receive enough blood flow and sustain good blood circulation, these two phases must be in harmony.

Understanding how different physiological processes interact is essential to understanding blood pressure regulation. The intricate regulation of blood pressure is facilitated by the renin-angiotensin-aldosterone system, the autonomic nervous system, and local variables within blood vessels. The complex nature of blood pressure homeostasis is highlighted by the fact that dysregulation of any one of these systems can result in hypertension.

High Blood Pressure Versus Normal:

Maintaining normal blood pressure guarantees that tissues and organs receive enough blood flow without overtaxing the circulatory system, which is crucial for general health. There are several levels of blood pressure, and the ideal blood pressure is less than 120/80 mmHg. Hypertension is the diagnosis made when a patient's blood pressure continuously falls above this level.

High blood pressure, often known as hypertension, is a serious health risk because it puts undue strain on the heart and may eventually damage arteries and organs. The illness is sometimes called the "silent killer" since it can worsen without any obvious signs. High blood pressure is caused by several factors, including age, genetics, lifestyle decisions (such as food and exercise), and underlying medical disorders.

Untreated hypertension has serious side effects that can include an elevated risk of stroke, heart disease, kidney damage, and other cardiovascular issues. Therefore, controlling and preventing hypertension requires routine blood pressure checks as well as lifestyle changes. Dietary modifications, more exercise, stress management techniques, and, in certain situations, medicines are examples of lifestyle modifications.

Hypertension affects every part of the circulatory system, with far-reaching effects on cardiovascular health. Atherosclerosis, a disorder marked by the accumulation of plaque in the arteries, can be brought on by the continuous, high stress exerted on arterial walls. A hazardous feedback loop is created when blood pressure rises and artery narrowing and hardening increase the risk of blood clots.

The heart, which pumps blood throughout the body, is put under a great deal of stress in people with hypertension. This may eventually cause the heart muscle to grow or hypertrophy, which would make it less effective. Heart failure, coronary artery disease, and other cardiovascular events are significantly increased by hypertension.

Moreover, blood arteries in vital organs including the kidneys and brain are directly threatened by hypertension. The enhanced risk of strokes and kidney disease can result from the harm caused by the increased pressure on small blood arteries. Thus, maintaining cardiovascular health requires understanding and controlling hypertension, underscoring the significance of early identification, prompt intervention, and preventive actions.

CHAPTER THREE

IDENTIFYING SYMPTOMS AND SIGNS
Silent Dangers: Unnoticed High Blood Pressure

Because hypertension, also referred to as high blood pressure, rarely causes any symptoms, it is frequently called a "silent killer". Asymptomatic hypertension refers to the possibility of high blood pressure in people who don't exhibit any symptoms. Since many people may not become aware of their condition until it reaches a critical stage or causes serious consequences, this silent threat can be misleading.

When hypertension first manifests, it can be difficult for people to identify it because of the lack of obvious symptoms. In contrast to certain medical conditions that have obvious warning indicators, hypertension works covertly, slowly damaging blood vessels, the heart, and other important organs. As a result, people may unintentionally maintain high blood pressure for a prolonged amount of time, raising their chance of developing severe cardiovascular conditions.

It is essential to regularly check blood pressure to diagnose asymptomatic hypertension. Regular examinations and screenings are crucial, particularly for those who have risk factors including a history of hypertension in their family, bad eating habits, sedentary lifestyles, or advanced age. The fact that asymptomatic hypertension is a thing now highlights how crucial it is to take preventative care of oneself and to see a doctor frequently to identify this silent threat before it worsens.

Recognizing Warning Indications and Symptoms

Even while hypertension is frequently asymptomatic, some people may experience specific indications and symptoms, particularly as the illness worsens. These symptoms may include headaches that don't go away, lightheadedness, dyspnea, and blurred vision. It's crucial to remember that these symptoms are not specific to hypertension and could also be linked to other medical conditions. But when these symptoms appear, they could be red flags that call for additional research, which could involve checking blood pressure and speaking with a medical expert.

Intense headaches are usually associated with hypertension, particularly in the morning. The cardiovascular system's strain may cause dizziness and lightheadedness by affecting blood flow to the brain. Breathlessness could be a sign that the heart is pumping blood more forcefully than usual, and vision issues could be the result of hypertensive damage to the blood vessels in the eyes.

These symptoms highlight how crucial it is to pay attention to one's body and consult a doctor if any unexpected symptoms are noticed. Early symptom diagnosis can result in prompt management and intervention, which may stop the course of hypertension and its related problems.

When to Get Medical Help

For prompt diagnosis and treatment of hypertension, it is essential to know when to seek medical help. It is advised to regularly check blood pressure, particularly in those who have risk factors. Medical treatment should be sought as soon as blood pressure readings routinely reveal levels above the normal range.

If you experience symptoms like intense headaches, chest pain, difficulty breathing, or changes in your vision, you should get medical help right away. These signs could point to a hypertensive crisis, which is a medical emergency that has to be treated right once to avoid more serious consequences like organ damage or stroke.

Even in the absence of symptoms, people with a family history of hypertension, older persons, and those with prior medical issues should continue to get regular checkups. Effective management of hypertension and lowering the risk of related problems depend heavily on proactive monitoring and early intervention.

By seeking medical attention when necessary, people may take charge of their health and collaborate with healthcare providers to create individualized blood pressure management plans.

CHAPTER FOUR

CHANGING YOUR LIFESTYLE TO CONTROL BLOOD PRESSURE
The Value of Nutritious Eating Practices

Eating well is essential for regulating blood pressure and enhancing cardiovascular health in general. Foods we eat have a direct impact on blood vessel function, weight control, and cholesterol levels. Consuming a diet high in fruits, vegetables, whole grains, lean meats, low-fat dairy products, and whole grains helps lower blood pressure and lowers the risk of the consequences of hypertension.

Controlling salt consumption is one of the most important factors in keeping blood pressure in a healthy range. Consuming too much salt can cause blood pressure to rise and fluid retention. As a result, it is advised that people consume less salt and favor fresh, unprocessed meals over packaged and processed ones. Incorporating foods high in potassium, such as oranges, bananas, and leafy greens, can also help control blood pressure and mitigate the negative effects of salt.

Moreover, there have been noteworthy improvements in blood pressure control demonstrated by implementing the DASH (Dietary Approaches to Stop Hypertension) eating plan. A balanced diet low in cholesterol, added sugars and saturated and trans fats is the focus of this strategy. People can positively affect their blood pressure and lower their risk of complications associated with hypertension by emphasizing nutrient-dense diets.

Guidelines for Physical Activity and Exercise:

One of the most important strategies for managing and preventing hypertension is regular physical activity. Exercise improves cardiovascular health, aids in maintaining ideal blood pressure levels, and helps with weight management. It has been demonstrated that resistance training and aerobic activity, such as jogging, cycling, or brisk walking, both lower blood pressure.

The American Heart Association suggests engaging in muscle-strengthening activities at least twice a week in addition to 150 minutes of moderate-intensity aerobic activity or 75 minutes of vigorous-intensity exercise per week. These recommendations encourage people to engage in long-term, enjoyable activities, which increases the likelihood that they will stick to a regular exercise schedule.

In addition to lowering blood pressure, exercise lowers the risk of heart disease and stroke, which enhances cardiovascular health overall. It also helps with weight management, which is essential for preventing hypertension. Frequent exercise stimulates blood vessel dilatation, improves blood flow, and supports the cardiovascular system's general health.

Techniques for Stress Management:

Stress plays a major role in high blood pressure, so controlling stress is essential to lowering blood pressure. Long-term stress can cause the release of hormones that raise heart rate and constrict blood vessels, which can eventually result in hypertension. Consequently, implementing stress-reduction strategies is crucial for maintaining cardiovascular health in general.

Mindfulness meditation is one method of stress management that is highly advised. This technique entails concentrating on the here and now, frequently by employing guided meditation exercises and deep breathing. Research has demonstrated that practicing mindfulness meditation helps lower blood pressure readings, both systolic and diastolic.

Beyond its cardiovascular advantages, regular exercise is also a highly effective stress reliever. The body's natural mood enhancers, endorphins, are released when exercise is performed and can help counteract the negative effects of stress. Incorporating mindfulness-based physical exercises like tai chi or yoga might be very beneficial for reducing stress.

Moreover, the establishment of constructive coping strategies, such as upholding a robust social support system, establishing achievable objectives, and giving precedence to leisure and relaxation periods, can make a substantial impact on stress mitigation. People can improve their blood pressure and general cardiovascular health by addressing stressors and implementing preventative measures.

CHAPTER FIVE

DRUGS AND ALTERNATIVE THERAPIES
Synopsis of Medicines for Hypertension

High blood pressure, or hypertension, is a chronic medical problem that needs to be managed thoroughly, and frequently with the help of medication. Effective treatment of hypertension requires an understanding of the many kinds of medicines.

Angiotensin-converting enzyme (ACE) inhibitors are a key class of drugs. These medications, which include lisinopril and enalapril, function by preventing the body from converting angiotensin I into angiotensin II, a strong vasoconstrictor. ACE inhibitors lower blood pressure by relaxing blood vessels in this way.

Angiotensin II receptor blockers (ARBs), which include valsartan and losartan, make up a different class. ARBs cause vasodilation and a drop in blood pressure by directly blocking the activity of angiotensin II at its receptors. Verapamil and amlodipine, two calcium channel blockers, are also frequently recommended. By preventing calcium from entering vascular smooth muscle cells, they increase vasodilation and reduce blood pressure.

Diuretics, such as furosemide and hydrochlorothiazide, are vital for controlling hypertension because they encourage the excretion of salt and fluids, which lowers blood volume and, in turn, blood pressure. Metoprolol and atenolol are examples of beta-blockers that lower heart rate and contractility, which help regulate blood pressure.

Patients who have certain comorbidities or resistant hypertension may be administered vasodilators, central agonists, or alpha-blockers. Alpha-blockers aid in blood vessel occlusion by relaxing specific muscles. By influencing the central nervous system, central agonists lessen blood vessel constriction. Vasodilators lower blood pressure by directly widening blood arteries. However, because of the possible negative effects, these drugs are frequently saved for particular situations.

It is crucial to remember that prescription drugs for hypertension may have adverse effects, and determining the best combination for a given person frequently necessitates careful observation and modifications. For long-term success in treating hypertension and avoiding consequences like heart disease and stroke, adherence to prescription regimens is essential.

Alternative Medicine

When it comes to the comprehensive management of hypertension, complementary therapies are invaluable adjuncts to traditional medical care. Alterations in lifestyle and alternative methods can improve general health and help regulate blood pressure.

First of all, a heart-healthy diet that emphasizes whole grains, fruits, vegetables, low-fat dairy products, and whole grains while limiting sodium intake is the

Dietary Approaches to Stop Hypertension (DASH) diet. By addressing lifestyle variables that contribute to hypertension, this nutritional strategy serves as a complement to medicine.

Frequent exercise is also another crucial adjunctive treatment. Exercise helps to maintain a healthy weight and strengthens the heart. Aerobic exercises, like cycling, swimming, or walking, have been demonstrated to lower blood pressure. Furthermore, stress-reduction methods like yoga, deep breathing exercises, and meditation can help lower hypertension brought on by stress.

A few dietary supplements, like those high in potassium, magnesium, and omega-3 fatty acids, may have a slight effect on controlling blood pressure. Before adding supplements to a program, it's important to speak with a healthcare provider, though, as they may interfere with prescriptions or have unexpected side effects.

Some people find that alternative therapies including massage therapy, biofeedback, and acupuncture help control their hypertension. These methods might provide further assistance for people looking for a more thorough treatment plan, even if research on their effectiveness is still being conducted.

Combining Medicine with Lifestyle Adjustments

A comprehensive strategy that incorporates lifestyle modifications is necessary for the effective management of hypertension in addition to medicines. Making changes to one's lifestyle can greatly increase the efficacy of prescription drugs, improving blood pressure regulation and cardiovascular health in general.

A key component of this integration is dietary adjustments. Because it lowers sodium intake and promotes heart health, the DASH diet—which is high in fruits, vegetables, lean proteins, and low-fat dairy—aligns with medication goals. Following this diet can improve the effectiveness of prescription drugs for hypertension.

Frequent exercise reduces stress, aids in weight loss, and enhances cardiovascular health in addition to medicine. Blood pressure can be considerably lowered by performing cardiovascular workouts for at least 150 minutes a week, as advised by health authorities.

Giving up smoking is a vital lifestyle modification for those with high blood pressure. In addition to immediately increasing blood pressure, smoking causes arterial stiffness and the emergence of cardiovascular disorders. Giving up smoking improves cardiovascular health in general as well as blood pressure control.

Another crucial component of combining medicine and lifestyle modifications is limiting alcohol use. Overindulgence in alcohol consumption can result in hypertension and can also affect how well antihypertensive drugs work. For those with high blood pressure, moderation or abstinence is advised.

Stress-reduction methods, such as yoga, meditation, and mindfulness, can be used in addition to medicine to treat the psychological causes of high blood pressure. Chronic stress can make hypertension worse, thus incorporating these methods into daily life will improve health in general.

In conclusion, a comprehensive strategy for controlling hypertension combines medicine with lifestyle modifications. Pharmacological therapies are more effective when combined with lifestyle adjustments that promote a healthier cardiovascular system, even if drugs target blood pressure directly. In addition to improving blood pressure control, this synergistic strategy lowers the risk of complications related to hypertension. People with hypertension must collaborate closely with medical specialists to create a customized treatment plan that combines medication and long-term lifestyle modifications.

CHAPTER SIX

AT-HOME BLOOD PRESSURE MONITORING AND MANAGEMENT
Selecting an Appropriate Blood Pressure Monitor:

Making an informed choice about a blood pressure monitor is an essential first step in managing hypertension at home. Monitors come in two primary varieties: automated and manual. More expertise and practice are needed for manual monitors, which use an inflatable arm cuff and a stethoscope. Conversely, automatic monitors are easy to operate and appropriate even for those without medical knowledge.

The cuff size is an important factor to take into account when selecting a blood pressure monitor. Inaccurate readings can arise from using the incorrect cuff size. The majority of monitors have adjustable cuffs, but it's important to make sure your arm fits correctly. Additionally, because of their accuracy and convenience of use, digital monitors are highly recommended. The whole monitoring experience can be improved by looking for features like multiple user memory and irregular heartbeat detection.

Choosing a monitor that has been approved by groups such as the British Hypertension Society (BHS) or the Association for the Advancement of Medical Instrumentation (AAMI) is a good idea. Validation guarantees that the monitor has undergone thorough accuracy testing. Lastly, it is wise to speak with a healthcare provider before buying a monitor because they may offer tailored advice based on each person's unique medical requirements.

Frequent Observation and Documentation:

One of the most important components of successful hypertension management is routine home blood pressure monitoring. Frequent blood pressure checks yield useful information that can help patients and medical professionals alike comprehend blood pressure trends and make wise decisions. Every day at the same time, monitoring should be done, and it's important to take precise readings by according to the prescribed recommendations.

To follow variations over time, a thorough record of blood pressure readings must be kept. Trends, triggers, and possible variations can be found by utilizing a digital health app or keeping a dedicated diary with the date, time, and readings. During doctor's appointments, these records become useful tools that help medical practitioners make well-informed changes to treatment programs.

Monitoring requires consistency, therefore people should make an effort to follow a schedule. Noting lifestyle factors in the record can provide further insights, as they might influence blood pressure. These aspects include stress, food, and physical activity. The documented information additionally promotes efficient correspondence with medical professionals, cultivating a cooperative strategy for the treatment of hypertension.

How to Interpret the Readings You've Done:

Accurate blood pressure interpretation is essential for making well-informed decisions on the management of hypertension. Systolic pressure, which is the upper number, and diastolic pressure, which is the lower number, make up a blood pressure reading. Generally speaking, a normal blood pressure value is 120/80 mm Hg. People who check their blood pressure at home must comprehend the meaning behind these figures.

High values can be a sign of hypertension, and they should be taken seriously right away if they persist. Understanding the recommendations' definitions of normal, high, and hypertensive values is critical. While a single high reading does not always point to an issue, recurrent increases should be explored with a medical practitioner.

It is equally crucial to interpret trends in blood pressure data. Modifications to lifestyle or treatment regimens can be based on long-term monitoring for consistent increases or declines. Recognizing these variables is crucial for optimal control of blood pressure because it can be impacted by a variety of factors, including stress, medication adherence, and lifestyle modifications.

It is crucial to have regular contact with medical professionals to analyze and act upon blood pressure data. To improve overall cardiovascular health, open communication guarantees that people receive timely counsel and modifications to their hypertension management strategy.

CHAPTER SEVEN

IMPORTANCE OF REGULAR CHECK-UPS
The Role of Healthcare Professionals:

Healthcare providers are essential in the fight against hypertension because they offer critical interventions and experienced assistance. High blood pressure, or hypertension, is a silent killer that frequently remains undiagnosed until serious problems occur. Frequent visits with medical professionals are necessary for the early identification, close observation, and efficient treatment of hypertension.

Doctors are the experts when it comes to treating hypertension; they use their training to identify risk factors, do in-depth exams, and recommend the right drugs. Due to the tight relationship between hypertension and cardiovascular problems, cardiologists, in particular, are experts in heart health and play a crucial role in managing cases of hypertension. In addition to diagnosing hypertension, these specialists counsel patients on lifestyle adjustments, such as dietary adjustments and exercise regimens, to support medicinal therapies.

Regular check-ups by nurses and other healthcare professionals play a major role in managing hypertension. They keep an eye on blood pressure, teach patients self-care techniques, and make sure that prescriptions are taken as directed. Furthermore, pharmacists are essential in medication management because they can provide advice on possible drug interactions and adverse effects, which improves patient safety in general.

Frequent communication with medical specialists helps to create individualized care plans that are specific to each patient's needs. These specialists evaluate how hypertension is developing, modify medication regimens as needed, and take care of any new health issues. Additionally, they provide patients with information that empowers them and promotes active engagement in their healthcare journey.

Frequent Examinations And Screenings For Health:

The mainstays of managing and preventing hypertension are routine examinations and screenings. Regular monitoring is important since it can identify hypertension early on and allow for prompt action to avoid consequences. Health screenings offer important information about a person's general state of health. These screenings frequently involve blood pressure checks, cholesterol checks, and glucose tests.

Regular check-ups enable medical practitioners to monitor changes in blood pressure over time, detecting trends and possible causes. For those who have risk factors like a family history of hypertension, bad lifestyle choices, or pre-existing medical issues, these checks are especially important. Regular check-ups enable early detection and rapid introduction of pharmaceutical and lifestyle adjustments, thereby significantly slowing the progression of hypertension.

Regular health examinations also help to prevent secondary hypertension-related consequences such as renal damage, heart disease, and stroke. Early detection of these risk factors reduces the overall burden of hypertension-related morbidity and mortality by enabling tailored therapies and lifestyle modifications.

Collaborative Care: Physician And Patient Collaboration:

Effective treatment of hypertension necessitates teamwork between medical providers and patients. This collaboration places a strong emphasis on collaborative decision-making and active participation, acknowledging that controlling hypertension is a lifetime commitment that goes beyond visiting a doctor's office.

Patients are essential to the collaborative care approach because they are major stakeholders in their health.

This entails keeping doctor's visits on time, being open and honest about symptoms and lifestyle choices, and actively following treatment regimens as directed. Patients need to follow doctor's orders on medication schedules, lifestyle changes, and at-home blood pressure monitoring.

Conversely, medical professionals encourage a cooperative atmosphere by teaching patients about hypertension, its effects, and the significance of following treatment regimens. To address any issues or obstacles that can prevent efficient hypertension control, they promote open communication. By ensuring that treatment plans reflect the preferences of the patient, shared decision-making enhances long-term adherence and overall patient engagement.

To sum up, the collaborative care approach highlights how patients and healthcare providers are intertwined in the fight against hypertension. Regular check-ups allow patients to actively participate in their care while healthcare professionals provide guidance and monitoring.

This synergy improves the efficacy of hypertension management techniques. To achieve optimal health outcomes and lessen the negative effects of hypertension on people's health as well as the health of the general public, collaboration is essential.

CHAPTER EIGHT

UNDERSTANDING THE RELATIONSHIPS BETWEEN OTHER HEALTH CONDITIONS AND HYPERTENSION
Heart Disease With Hypertension:

Understanding the complex link between cardiac disease and hypertension is essential to comprehend the many facets of hypertension. High blood pressure, or hypertension, is a major factor in the emergence and advancement of several cardiovascular diseases, the most serious of which is heart disease. An extended period of high blood pressure puts an undue amount of strain on the heart and damages the cardiovascular system.

As the main organ in charge of pumping blood throughout the body, the heart is directly impacted by high blood pressure. The heart's muscles stiffen as a result of the increased pressure, which makes the heart work harder to pump blood. This disorder, called left ventricular hypertrophy, is frequently brought on by hypertension and is linked to a higher risk of heart failure. Moreover, the accumulation of plaque in the arteries caused by atherosclerosis is a condition that is exacerbated by hypertension. Because atherosclerosis obstructs blood flow, heart attacks and other cardiac events are more likely to occur.

Furthermore, coronary artery disease (CAD), a disorder in which the blood arteries supplying the heart narrow or block, is significantly increased by hypertension. The likelihood of suffering a myocardial infarction (heart attack) is greatly increased when high blood pressure and atherosclerosis coexist. Understanding the relationship between hypertension and heart disease is critical since controlling blood pressure is the first line of defense against the damaging effects on the cardiovascular system.

Effects on the Kidneys:

The complex relationship that exists between kidney health and hypertension emphasizes how important blood pressure control is to preserving ideal renal function. One of the main causes of chronic kidney disease (CKD) is hypertension, and the kidneys are particularly susceptible to the negative consequences of high blood pressure. Because of the complex web of blood veins in the kidneys, they are especially vulnerable to variations in blood pressure, and chronic hypertension can lead to nephron damage.

The constant strain placed on the fragile nephrons, the kidney's filtration units, can result in weakened waste elimination and blood filtration. This can eventually lead to chronic kidney disease and renal dysfunction over time. Furthermore, high blood pressure quickens the course of pre-existing kidney diseases, increasing the likelihood of end-stage renal disease (ESRD) and requiring more extensive treatments like dialysis or kidney transplantation.

Understanding that the relationship is reciprocal is crucial because renal failure can also exacerbate hypertension. Through its ability to control blood volume and electrolyte levels, the kidneys are essential in maintaining blood pressure regulation. The body may retain more sodium when kidney function deteriorates, which could result in fluid retention and elevated blood pressure. This complex interaction highlights the necessity of comprehensive approaches to hypertension management to protect renal health.

Connection to Other Conditions and Diabetes:

The complex relationship between high blood pressure and diabetes as well as other medical disorders emphasizes the systemic effects of high blood pressure on several physiological functions. Diabetes makes people more prone to hypertension, which poses a serious combined risk that greatly increases the likelihood of cardiovascular problems. Diabetes can worsen the effects of hypertension on the cardiovascular system by affecting blood vessel function and accelerating the atherosclerotic processes.

Moreover, there is a close relationship between hypertension and metabolic syndrome, a group of disorders that includes aberrant lipid profiles, high blood pressure, raised blood sugar, and abdominal obesity. The chance of acquiring type 2 diabetes, cardiovascular disease, and other associated conditions is greatly increased by this syndrome. Therefore, treating hypertension is essential to controlling and delaying the development of metabolic syndrome.

It's also important to recognize the connection between cerebrovascular illnesses like strokes and hypertension. High blood pressure increases the risk of hemorrhagic or ischemic strokes by damaging the fragile blood vessels in the brain. Controlling high blood pressure is essential to lower the chance of these catastrophic brain occurrences.

Finally, to create comprehensive strategies to counteract the negative consequences of raised blood pressure on the body, it is imperative to comprehend the complex relationships that exist between hypertension and heart disease, kidney health, diabetes, and other illnesses.

To treat hypertension holistically and ultimately improve general health and well-being, blood pressure must be regulated in addition to its effects on different organs and systems.

CHAPTER NINE

NUTRITIONAL STRATEGIES FOR CONTROLLING BLOOD PRESSURE
The DASH Diet's Advantages

One notable pillar in the treatment of hypertension is the Dietary Approaches to Stop Hypertension (DASH) diet. The DASH diet, created by the National Heart, Lung, and Blood Institute, places a strong emphasis on eating a balanced, heart-healthy diet. Its main tenets include limiting sodium consumption, eating a range of foods high in nutrients, and encouraging moderation in total calorie intake. With a wealth of evidence to support it, the DASH diet is well known for its ability to effectively control blood pressure.

The DASH diet's emphasis on fruits and vegetables is one of its main tenets. Essential vitamins, minerals, and antioxidants included in these foods support cardiovascular health as a whole. The diet also suggests including low-fat dairy items, lean meats, and whole grains. These components guarantee a balanced dietary profile that promotes ideal blood pressure levels.

Limiting salt intake is a key component of the DASH diet. Because high sodium intake is associated with high blood pressure, the DASH diet promotes a lower salt intake to address this issue. Putting more focus on whole, fresh meals rather than processed and packaged goods encourages people to naturally consume less salt. Not only does this dietary strategy work well for controlling hypertension, but it also supports other health objectives like controlling weight and preventing other cardiovascular diseases.

Studies have repeatedly shown how beneficial the DASH diet is. Research indicates that people who follow the DASH guidelines have significant drops in their blood pressure, both in the systolic and diastolic values. Additionally, the diet has been linked to better lipid profiles and a lower chance of heart disease. These results highlight the DASH diet's long-term beneficial effects on general cardiovascular health.

To sum up, the DASH diet is a thorough and scientifically supported method of controlling hypertension through dietary decisions. It is an effective technique for promoting heart health and lowering the risk of cardiovascular diseases because it places a strong emphasis on nutrient-rich foods, moderation in calorie intake, and sodium restriction.

Suggested Dietary Adjustments

It takes a comprehensive approach to dietary decisions to manage hypertension with food; it is not enough to simply follow a certain diet. In addition to the DASH diet, several other suggested dietary modifications are vital for controlling blood pressure.

It is imperative to give foods high in potassium priority. A diet high in potassium can help lower blood pressure because it counteracts the effects of salt on blood pressure. Foods high in potassium, like potatoes, bananas, oranges, and leafy greens, ought to be included in every day's meals.

Cutting back on saturated and trans fats is another significant nutritional adjustment. These fats have the potential to cause hypertension and a higher risk of heart disease by contributing to the accumulation of cholesterol in the arteries. Limiting red meat and processed meals and consuming lean protein sources like fish, chicken, lentils, and nuts will help maintain heart health and control blood pressure.

Moreover, consuming more fiber in your diet helps control your blood pressure. Whole grains, fruits, vegetables, legumes, and other diets high in fiber have been linked to lowered blood pressure. Fiber contributes to weight management, which is an essential component of controlling hypertension, by regulating blood sugar levels and encouraging a sensation of fullness.

Reducing alcohol intake is another suggested dietary adjustment. Excessive alcohol use can cause blood pressure to rise, even while moderate alcohol consumption may have cardiovascular benefits.

Depending on their health, people with hypertension should either limit their alcohol use to moderate amounts or abstain from it completely.

All things considered, these suggested dietary adjustments support the DASH diet's tenets and offer a thorough approach to blood pressure control. People can improve the efficacy of their dietary strategy for hypertension by including foods high in potassium, cutting back on trans and saturated fats, increasing their intake of fiber, and consuming alcohol in moderation.

Recipes for Heart-Healthy Dinners

Making heart-healthy meals is essential to controlling hypertension, and using the appropriate cooking methods can help a lot with this. Cooking techniques that emphasize nutrient retention over the use of harmful fats and excess sodium are essential for preserving cardiovascular health.

Using techniques that entail the least amount of extra fat is one of the most important cooking recommendations for heart-healthy meals. As great substitutes for deep-frying or overusing butter and lard when cooking, tiny amounts of heart-healthy oils can be used for grilling, baking, steaming, and sautéing. These techniques remove extraneous calories and unhealthy fats from food while maintaining its natural flavors and nutritional value.

Another key component of heart-healthy cooking is using a variety of herbs and spices. Herbs and spices give food more depth and complexity than salt does, all without increasing the amount of sodium consumed. This is especially important for people who are on the DASH diet, which stresses lowering salt intake. Adding flavors to food using spices like cumin and turmeric and herbs like thyme, rosemary, and basil can improve the flavor of food without sacrificing its heart-healthy qualities.

When cooking for heart health, choosing lean proteins and including plant-based protein sources are crucial factors to take into account. Reducing the amount of saturated fat consumed can be achieved by choosing skinless chicken, fish, lentils, and tofu over fatty meat cuts. Moreover, incorporating a range of vibrant veggies into meals guarantees a varied assortment of vital nutrients in addition to adding aesthetic appeal.

For people who are controlling their hypertension, cutting back on processed and pre-packaged foods is an essential cooking guideline. These foods frequently have high salt and bad fat content. People can better regulate how much sodium they eat and customize dishes to fit their nutritional objectives when they cook with fresh, whole ingredients.

In summary, implementing heart-healthy cooking techniques is an essential part of a comprehensive blood pressure control plan. People can prioritize their cardiovascular health while still enjoying great meals by selecting lean proteins, adding flavor with herbs and spices, cooking methods that preserve nutritious content, and avoiding processed foods.

CHAPTER TEN

OVERCOMING OBSTACLES AND MAINTAINING DRIVE
Typical Barriers to the Management of Hypertension:

Managing hypertension presents several obstacles that people must overcome to effectively control their blood pressure. One frequent challenge is finding it difficult to follow a regular regimen for taking medications. Due to forgetfulness, adverse effects, or the conviction that they can manage their illness without medicine, many people find it difficult to take their medications regularly. A tailored strategy is needed to overcome this barrier, one that includes clearing up any misunderstandings and educating people on the significance of prescription drugs.

The influence of lifestyle factors on blood pressure is another barrier. Stress, insufficient exercise, and unhealthy eating patterns can all lead to high blood pressure. Although it might be challenging to break old habits and embrace a healthier lifestyle, doing so is essential for managing hypertension. To address these issues, a thorough treatment strategy can include nutrition counseling, consistent exercise regimens, and stress-reduction strategies.

Furthermore, a lot of people struggle financially, which makes it difficult for them to get essential medical care or buy prescription drugs. Investigating affordable alternatives, such as generic drugs, government aid programs, or neighborhood services, may be necessary to get past this barrier. Support systems and healthcare providers are essential in helping people get over these financial difficulties.

Putting Together a Support Network:

Creating a strong support network is essential to overcoming hypertension throughout the path. People dealing with this physical issue frequently carry emotional and psychological weights, and a support network can offer the necessary understanding and encouragement. Important members of this support system include friends, family, and medical professionals.

Family involvement is especially important since they may help with medication adherence, actively participate in lifestyle improvements, and offer emotional support. Educating family members about hypertension improves their comprehension and encourages teamwork in the management of the illness.

Additionally, by offering knowledgeable counsel, keeping track of developments, and modifying treatment plans as necessary, medical experts make a substantial contribution to the support system. Strong support systems are built through frequent check-ups, honest communication, and a cooperative attitude between patients and healthcare professionals.

Peer support groups can also be helpful since they provide people the chance to talk about their experiences, trade coping mechanisms, and get inspiration from others going through comparable struggles. By fostering a sense of community, these organizations help people feel less alone and give them the confidence to take an active role in managing their hypertension.

Sustaining Motivation Over Time:

Maintaining motivation over the long haul is essential to managing hypertension successfully. A prevalent obstacle is the initial spurt of motivation, which may gradually fade. People need to celebrate little triumphs along the road and set realistic, achievable goals to address this. This method not only raises spirits but also supports the notion that managing hypertension is an ongoing process.

Additionally, adding fun activities to the routine might increase its sustainability and level of engagement. Engaging in interesting hobbies, socializing with others, and engaging in regular physical activity all enhance general well-being and sustain the urge to lead a healthy lifestyle.

Education is essential for maintaining motivation since it raises awareness of the long-term effects of hypertension and the advantages of continued treatment. People who comprehend the reasoning for dietary modifications and medication compliance are more likely to maintain their motivation in their fight against hypertension.

To sum up, developing a strong support network, eliminating typical barriers to hypertension management, and sustaining motivation over the long term are all interrelated components of a holistic strategy to overcome hypertension. Using a combination of medical, social, and psychological elements, this comprehensive approach gives people the ability to take charge of their health and strive for ideal blood pressure regulation.

CHAPTER ELEVEN

UPCOMING DEVELOPMENTS AND INNOVATIONS IN THE TREATMENT OF HYPERTENSION
Progress in the Field of Medicine:

Discoveries in the field of medicine have greatly advanced our knowledge of hypertension and opened the door to creative new methods of treating it. The finding of genetic markers linked to the risk of hypertension is one noteworthy development. Certain genes and genetic variations have been identified by researchers as being involved in the regulation of blood pressure. This information makes personalized medicine possible by enabling medical professionals to customize treatment regimens according to a patient's genetic profile.

Moreover, advances in pharmacogenomics have facilitated the creation of more precise and potent hypertension drugs.

Healthcare practitioners can prescribe drugs that are more likely to be effective and have fewer side effects by taking into account a patient's genetic composition. This signifies a move in the therapy of hypertension toward precision medicine, wherein therapies are tailored to the specific biological traits of each patient.

The investigation of new therapeutic targets is a noteworthy field of advancement. New medications with better safety and efficacy characteristics are being developed as a result of research into novel pathways and molecules involved in blood pressure regulation. Furthermore, novel therapeutic approaches have become possible due to the increased attention being paid to the gut microbiota and how it affects cardiovascular health. One such approach is the possible use of probiotics to lower blood pressure.

Technological developments in diagnostics and medical imaging have also improved our capacity to evaluate cardiovascular health. Early identification of hypertensive heart disease is facilitated by non-invasive imaging techniques like magnetic resonance imaging (MRI) and three-dimensional echocardiography, which offer comprehensive insights into the anatomy and function of the heart. Early identification makes it possible to implement more focused and proactive therapies, which eventually improves patient outcomes.

In summary, the field of hypertension management is undergoing a revolution due to continuous advancements in medical research, which include genetic discoveries, novel therapeutic targets, and advanced diagnostic technologies. These advancements open the door to more individualized and successful treatment plans while also expanding our knowledge of the fundamental mechanisms driving hypertension.

The Use of Technology in Monitoring Blood Pressure:

Technological advancements in blood pressure monitoring and treatment are revolutionizing the way individuals and healthcare professionals handle hypertension. The growing use of wearable technology for continuous blood pressure monitoring is one of the most noteworthy technological developments. Real-time monitoring of blood pressure throughout the day is made possible by smartwatches and other wearable sensors that are integrated with photoplethysmography (PPG) technology. This allows for a more dynamic and comprehensive picture of a person's cardiovascular health.

These wearables' accessibility and ease of use enable people to take an active role in managing their hypertension. In addition to helping identify aberrant blood pressure patterns early on, continuous monitoring enables a more sophisticated knowledge of the variables impacting blood pressure variability, such as stress, sleep, and physical exercise. Healthcare providers will be able to use this data to make more educated decisions and create individualized treatment programs.

Additionally, telemedicine has shown to be an effective method for controlling blood pressure, particularly in rural or underdeveloped areas.

Healthcare professionals may remotely track their patients' blood pressure readings and modify treatment plans as necessary thanks to remote patient monitoring platforms that are coupled with wireless blood pressure monitors. This increases patient involvement and lessens the need for routine in-person visits, improving accessibility and convenience of healthcare.

The analysis of the massive volumes of data produced by continuous blood pressure monitoring heavily relies on artificial intelligence (AI) and machine learning techniques. These technologies can recognize trends, anticipate episodes of hypertension, and provide personalized risk factor information. Healthcare professionals can improve long-term outcomes for people with hypertension by utilizing AI to move toward more proactive and preventive therapies.

In summary, the use of technology in blood pressure monitoring is transforming the management of hypertension by offering continuous, real-time data, improving patient involvement, and utilizing artificial intelligence to deliver more individualized and proactive care.

Potential Strategies for Preventing Hypertension:

The field of hypertension prevention is changing, moving toward more all-encompassing and individualized methods that take into account underlying physiological mechanisms as well as lifestyle factors. Investigating novel lifestyle therapies that go beyond conventional advice is one intriguing direction. Exercise prescriptions that are tailored to a person's fitness level, interests, and health are becoming more and more popular. These customized workout programs take into account variables like exercise type, duration, and intensity to maximize cardiovascular benefits and encourage adherence.

There is a paradigm change occurring in the dietary practices used to prevent hypertension. A greater focus is being placed on customized nutrition, which takes into account metabolic profile, genetic characteristics, and individual dietary sensitivities, in addition to generic principles. Precision nutrition, which customizes food plans based on each person's particular needs, has potential benefits for improving blood pressure regulation and cardiovascular health in general.

There will soon be breakthroughs in pharmaceutical prevention in addition to lifestyle therapies. New pharmacological discoveries focus on certain pathways linked to hypertension, offering alternatives to people who might not react well to conventional antihypertensive drugs. This includes drugs that target inflammation, adjust salt balance more skillfully, or modify the gut microbiota, creating new opportunities for preventative pharmacotherapy.

Additionally, the effectiveness of behavioral therapies and digital health tools together is improving tactics for preventing hypertension. People can encourage healthy behaviors by using real-time feedback, education, and support from mobile applications and virtual health platforms. The relevance of behavioral therapies in preventing and reducing hypertension is becoming more widely acknowledged. One example of such an intervention is cognitive-behavioral therapy for stress management.

The prevention of hypertension through a patient-centered, holistic approach is becoming more and more popular. To do this, preventive interventions must take into account the social determinants of health, which include socioeconomic factors and environmental impacts. To promote healthy behaviors and lower the overall burden of hypertension, communities, legislators, and healthcare providers must work together.

In summary, tailored and multimodal strategies that incorporate cutting-edge lifestyle treatments, precision nutrition, pharmaceutical advancements, and digital health tools will be key to preventing hypertension in the future. These innovative approaches have the potential to greatly reduce the worldwide burden of hypertension and enhance cardiovascular health on a population scale by targeting each person's unique needs and characteristics.

www.ingramcontent.com/pod-product-compliance
Lightning Source LLC
Chambersburg PA
CBHW050744260726
48661CB00001B/403